Still

Striving

The Testimony of
Barbara Shuler

An Autobiography

Still

Striving

The Testimony of
Barbara Shuler

An Autobiography

WRITE YOUR STORY PUBLISHING

Write Your Story Publishing, GLO LLC
920 Haddonfield Road #716
Cherry Hill, NJ 08002

Barbara Shuler

Still Striving: The Testimony of Barbara Shuler, An Autobiography. *Copyright ©2020 Barbara Shuler.*

WYS books may be ordered through booksellers or bulk orders may be fulfilled by contacting the author or:
WYS Publishing, formerly GLO Publishing
https://www.glotap.org
gloinc2015@gmail.com
1-609-784-9698

ISBN: 978-1-7342821-3-9 (Paperback Edition)

BIO002010   BIO026000   BIO022000   BIO038000   BIO033000

Printed in the United States of America
WYS Publishing date: July 2020

Write Your Story Publishing, GLO LLC
920 Haddonfield Road #716
Cherry Hill, NJ 08002

Introduction

Every able child has dreams. Some of those dreams change, while others remain the same. For me, my dream was the same from the time I was just six years old. My dream was to become a nurse.

I began learning necessary skills, as I babysat children. In New York, this dream began to have more focus, as my passion developed into the desire to help children. I worked at a place called "The Foundling Home," and there is where I knew just how much I wanted to help children.

My church, where my spiritual life has grown, gave me the opportunity to direct this passion by serving as President of the Children's Church Ministry. Even when I was not in charge, I taught Sunday School and helped others.

My dream to become a nurse was also fulfilled. I became a nurse and so enjoyed my role! Even at the age of 67, I still loved crafts, teaching, and going with my Sunday School children to visit the sick. My dad taught school, so teaching was in my blood.

After 43 years enjoying life as a nurse, tragedy struck.

~~~~~~

My Story

∽1960∾

January 14
Dear Diary, My mother's birthday is today. I had a nice time in school today.

January 24
Dear Diary, Today, I went to a Grapefruit Tea at our church and had a wonderful time!

February 13
Dear Diary, Today, I was very disappointed because it snowed, and the choir I am in could not have our anniversary.

March 2
Dear Diary, Today, it snowed again. We got out of school at 1:00.

March 6

Dear Diary, Today was my brother's birthday. This is the first time that I can remember celebrating his birthday without him getting a present.

March 9

Dear Diary, It snowed again today, and we did not go to school. I hate not going to school.

March 15

Dear Diary, Today is my birthday. My grandmother gave me a dollar! My mother is going to bake me a cake!

March 17

Dear Diary, We went back to school again. I had plenty of homework to do. George gave me a nickel.

March 26

Dear Diary, Today is Saturday. I rode my bike over to my aunt's house on 15th street.

April 18

Dear Diary, Today, I went to the church and got some eggs for Easter Monday. I also helped my daddy wax his car.

April 24

Today is my brother's birthday.

June 4

Dear Diary, Today, we went to school on a Saturday. I got promoted to the 10th grade!

June 8

Dear Diary, Today, I went over to Adele's, my aunt's house.

July 9

Dear Diary, Today, my friends from New York came to visit.

July 10

Dear Diary, I went to church. My friends got in trouble for going off.

Barbara Shuler

July 27

Dear Diary, My admirer called me! It was Connie Shuler! I'm so happy and excited!

August 4

Dear Diary, Today, Lacy B hugged me around my waist. Darius said he liked me. I like him.

August 7

Dear Diary, Today, I got baptized.

December 26

Dear Diary, After Christmas, I rode my bike.

This is also the year I got a polio vaccine.

৵1961৵

March 2

Dear Diary, Today, Reginald did not call, but that's okay. George O'Neal called me.

March 15

Dear Diary, Today is my birthday. I got a cake and a 50¢. I am Sweet 16 and have only been kissed once.

April 15

Dear Diary, My mother and father were fussing over a girl named, Fannie.

Reginald called and asked if he could have one of my pictures.

May 22

Dear Diary, I caught the measles and had to stay home.

June 27

Dear Diary, Today, my daddy got mad at me. He slapped me. Sometimes, I think I hate him. He says I sit around and talk. He never lets me go anywhere, and he scares my friends away by not being nice to them.

July 2
Dear Diary, Today, I went to a pie walk and won a pie!

July 10
Dear Diary, I am on my way to New York City today.

July 13
Dear Diary, Today, I went to Coney Island and had a wonderful time!

August 7
Dear Diary, My mother came to New York, too.

❧1962❧

March 15

Dear Diary, Today is my 17th birthday. I had a surprise birthday party!

May 13

Dear Diary, Reginald took me to the prom. I had a wonderful time! He kissed me good night!

June 4

Dear Diary, I went on a hayride to Martinsville, Virginia. Reginald ignored me.

November 1

I had the chicken pox.

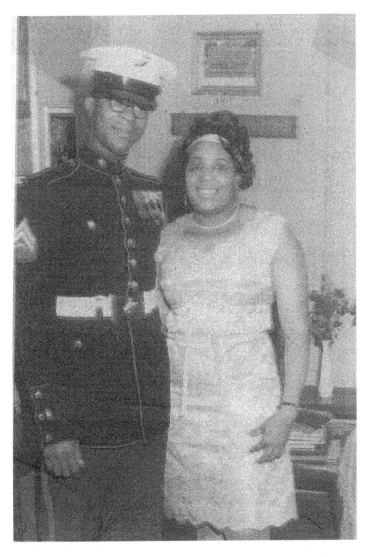

*1966- Barbara and Connie dressed for Lily's wedding.
The dress was light purple. I made it.*

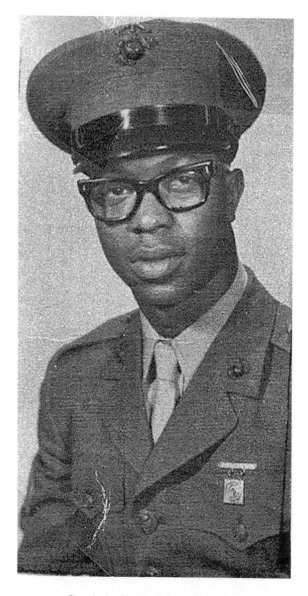

Connie in the Marines, 1965 - 1969

❧**1995**❧

March 15

I am 50 years old! Can you believe it?!

❧**1996**❧

January 14

My mother is 70 years old today. The "Blizzard of '96" is almost over.

March 9

My parents celebrated their 50th wedding anniversary. It was a wonderful, spiritual celebration. My brother, Man, couldn't make it. He is in jail in Arkansas.

March 15

I am 51 years old today! I had a wonderful birthday! I went out to eat and got presents from Adele Harris and my coworkers!

∽1998∾

March 9

It's snowing, while I'm at work on the evening shift. This is the first time in years!

∽2000∾

January 14

My mother is 74 years old today. She is very sick.

January 24

It's snowing, while I'm at work at 7:30 PM. I love it!

January 29

It snowed again! We got around five to six inches!

January 30

It's been sleeting all day. My mom is doing okay. My dad is her caretaker. On my day off, I'm over there a lot. My life is not my own. They have become my children. I do what I can for them.

❧**2001**☙

January 14

This is my mom's 75th birthday! We didn't think she would live from 2000. The doctor had told us there was nothing he could do. One year later, here she is, still with us. To God be the glory! We celebrated with a party at Ron's Hotel.

Some of those present were:

Husband, Alonzo; son, Ronald; Ron's wife, Alesia; daughter, Barbara; grandchildren: Todd (Barbara's son) and Ron Jr (Ron's son); great-grandchildren: Fred, Chris, Kim, and Jerome. The great-grands are Kima's (Ron's daughter's) children.

This was a very special time!

January 23

I'm off work today. My mom has been feeling good. Today, I am over at their house because my dad needs some time to do some things.

So, I ate breakfast, hemmed his pants, dusted, looked at a craft book, cooked, ate lunch, and took a nap.

January 27

I had a very busy day. We spent the day at one of my friend's son's funeral. He was only 17. He died of meningitis. It was sad, but the funeral was very uplifting. Elder Curry's sermon was entitled, "Touch Down."

February 4

I worked this Sunday but got off early. Our connection group went to visit David Rozier. He uplifted us instead of us uplifting him. The group today included: Phyllis and Jonathan Stewart, Pat Howard, Liz Maxwell and me.

December 27

My mother went into the hospital Monday morning. It was Christmas Eve. She should have gone last Friday, but she didn't want to. I think she knew it would be her last time, so she did not want to leave the house. She and Dad even pushed themselves to go to church Sunday, but she had to leave early.

Guess what? My brother, Ronnie, had asked her what she wanted. Her only response was, "Barbara needs a car."

Mommy was in so much agony those two hours. She said to me, "Barbara, you don't know how I feel. I think I'll go on and die."

I didn't answer her because I didn't know what to say. I just rubbed her back and her head. When the hospital staff couldn't get a reading for her blood pressure, I knew it was the end.

Mommy went to be with her Lord tonight, between 8:30 and 9:00 PM. She stayed warm, until we all had talked to her and told her we understood that she was tired and to do what she needed to do.

Bye, Mommy. Thanks for loving me unconditionally. Thanks for taking care of and raising my son.

I love you,

Barbara.

Mom died a peaceful death. I only hope, in my lifetime, that I can be the strong woman she was.

December 28, 6:45 AM

Mommy missed her birthday by 18 days. Isn't it funny how the nurse who took care of her was named "Barbara," and the nurse's husband's name was "Todd"? God is good!

December 31, 2:00 PM

Mommy's funeral was today. She looked so good. She had on a winter white suit trimmed in brown velvet, lace gloves and a winter white hat. *I think she winked at me.*

My brother, Man, was there. Today was the first time we have seen him in, at least, ten years or more. He looked so sad and alone, as if he didn't belong with us.

Mom had a wonderful funeral. Elder Curry's sermon title was "And the Winner Is . . .!" It was so uplifting! The church served us dinner.

Ron's wife, Lisa, was great in helping to plan the funeral. We were able to get almost all of Man's family there.

A lot of my co-workers came to the wake.

∝2002∝

January 4, 12:00 A.M.

I'm sad tonight. . . Well, I guess it's morning now. Yesterday was a week since Mommy died. It snowed, and I thought about the snow being on her, but I know her soul has already gone to Heaven. I can hear her talking to me and laughing.

It's another year, and there is still no one special in my life.

March 1

Today, I am very sad. I miss my Mommy today. During communion, for the first time, I really missed my mom. I cried and cried.

March 14

Today, Priscillia, from my job, took me to the movies to see *John Q*. This was my birthday present! Thank you!

March 15

Today is my birthday. This is my first birthday without my mom. My best friends, Liz and Pat, took me out to dinner at White Oak. I had a wonderful time!

Joy gave me a little party at work and a jacket. Betsy gave me towels. These two nurse friends have really helped me through my grief.

My brother and his wife, Ron and Lisa, were wonderful to me! I got two uniforms and some lace to make handkerchiefs.

Thanks, Mom, for making me love my birthday!

✑**2005**✑

January 14

Today is my mom's birthday, but she is no longer with us. She died in 2001. I miss her so much.

January 30

It's sleeting today. My mom and dad are both dead. I miss them a lot.

✑**2007**✑

May 3, 12:30 PM

I'm back at Wesley Long Hospital again after a year. The doctor saw two spots on my right lung. I had a CAT scan, and now, today, I'm getting a PET scan. I'm very nervous, and I'm almost in tears.

May 15

I will get a biopsy on May 24th. Everything will be good because I believe in God, and I believe everything will be okay. I have so much still to do.

❦**2009**❧

August 20

I have started school. I am going for my Master's Degree to become a Christian Counselor. I have not been studying for a long time. I spend most of my time in the Bible.

October 15

The semester is over. I earned an "A."

❦**2012**❧

In November, my life, as I knew it, changed forever.

It was the Thanksgiving holiday, and we were visiting my niece and her grandchildren. I sat down for a few minutes, while the family was taking pictures.

I remember one of the children asking, "Miss Barbara, are you sleepy?"

I recall replying, "Yes." My head was wobbling around, and then, I must have passed out.

They brought me a pillow and a blanket. To my surprise, my left hand and foot started shaking uncontrollably.

I yelled, "Go and get your Uncle Connie!"

When he came to take me to the hospital, I could not walk to the door which was only a few feet away. I was so frightened! He put me in the back seat of the car and headed to Greensboro.

On the way back, I asked him to stop at a gas station with a bathroom. He could not get me out of the car! I could not stand! I didn't know what was happening to me, and I was afraid, worried, and neither of us knew what to do! Getting back in the car, Connie hurried towards Greensboro!

As I lay in the back seat, I could feel the numbness traveling up my leg. I was holding a cup, as I started to pray. I asked God to stop the numbness, so it would not reach my hand. I prayed that my hand would not be deformed.

Then, my God intervened. He placed a deer in front of the car. The impact deployed the air bags, but we were not hurt. OnStar responded immediately, and an ambulance was dispatched.

If we had continued to Greensboro, I might not have survived. I had a stroke, which paralyzed my entire left side. You see, the deer lost its life so that mine could be saved.

❧**2013**☙

March 15
I am 68 years old today.

❧**2014**☙

November 26
Ms. Smile-a-Lot was not feeling well. She was even crying. I noticed a lot of my ACE friends are getting fragile. Ms. D.D., who can't hear, sounds like she has COPD from years of smoking. She makes sounds when sitting and breathing.

At the center, we had our Thanksgiving dinner. It was good. Taylor did a good job. We had potato salad, green bean casserole, sweet potatoes, dressing, ham, turkey, rolls, pumpkin pie, sweet potato pie, tea, and soda. Taylor is a very compassionate person.

I am walking stronger. It's getting closer to the anniversary of my stroke.

⊰**2015**⊱

September 18
Taylor took us, the ACE group, to the Greek Festival. It was fun to be with friends. Thank you, Taylor, for our outing.

I had a flashback! I rode on the ramp to get on the bus. Guess what? I was at the back of the bus, while all the white clients were "up front." I felt like I was in W—S, my childhood!

September 19
I went to a workshop on spiritual gifts. This is the second time I found out what my spiritual gifts are. It was an exciting seminar! Pastor Shark reminds me of Pastor Curry.

November 14

I am special! My 91-year-old aunt came to visit me! I was so excited, I cried. Paulette and Pebbles brought her. They talked openly about her cancer and pending death.

November 20, 6:00 AM

We started on our way to South Carolina to Connie's boyhood friend's funeral. We watched a beautiful sunrise! Then, we had said our prayer for traveling mercy.

Today was such a beautiful, fall day. The trees were so colorful. Connie explained that the magnificent, red trees were most likely maple trees. He's a country boy. We saw two black animals on the side of the road—maybe foxes?

While riding through the country, I was thinking about our forefathers. They must have had hard lives.

By 8:25 AM, we were passing over a river, and swamps were everywhere! Then, I could understand the song, "Swamp Fox." They had to have a scout to find dry land because they could not walk through all the water.

Wise men still seek him.

How did they get across the Santee River back then?

We started listening to Christmas songs in the car.

11:00 A.M. – The funeral was a nice service. The preacher preached from Matthew 24:1-7, "He is Coming Back."

I didn't go to the gravesite. There was too much dirt, and it required too much walking in the dirt.

Saturday after Thanksgiving will mark three years since I had my stroke and came back to St. George. Thank You, God, for my blessings and health! I have another chance to see the sunshine! Thank You, Jesus!

3:00 PM – We stopped by his friend's sister's house. I did not go in because there were steps, and I was tired. I was happy to just sit in the car. It was okay. I wanted him to visit as long as he wanted.

We also stopped at this white couple's house where my husband used to live. The woman who was living there was the sister of the man that my husband stayed with as a child. They were very hospitable, nice and very talkative.

I peed in my pamper because there was no bathroom.

November 26

This is my third year as a stroke victim. I have come so far. I testified as to God's blessings for the first time since my stroke back in South Carolina.

December 29

I have been in a funk and could not figure out why. It came to me about 6:00 tonight. My mom died December 27, 2001. Can you believe she has been gone away from me for 14 years?! Now, I know why I was feeling so down.

❧2016❧

January 14

We've crossed over into a new year!

Miss Betty Jo is leaving to go stay with her daughter in South Carolina. Miss Faye is going to Henry Street.

January 30

We're in the midst of a snow storm. It looks like the one we had in 2000! It sleeted all day today, just like it did yesterday.

⤙2020⤚

Today, I walk with a walker, and my Occupational Therapist has said my attention span is about 20 minutes. This stroke has stopped me from teaching my beloved Children's Church and helping with the Church Safety team.

You see, I had been a nurse for 43 years. Now, the paper had turned. For the first time, I wasn't helping others. I had to be helped. My kids have learned to help me: when I forget a word, they fill in the blank; when I have to go from the basement to the main sanctuary, we don't have an elevator but lots of stairs that I can't climb, so they've pushed me in a wheel chair; when I need help standing up or getting into a car, they support me.

This stroke has been a humbling experience, but because of my faith in God and the power of prayer, I am growing stronger each day, and like our church's mission statement, I will continue to "Strive for Excellence in Ministry."

About the Author

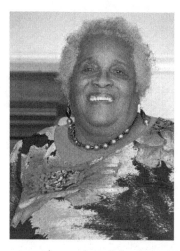

Barbara McCullough Shuler is a native of North Carolina who grew up in the midst of segregation. In the 60s, she went to the 1st integrated Nursing School in Winton Salem, NC. A few years later, she went back to college and received a BA in Mental Health. Barbara has held several nursing jobs but was an addiction nurse for 30 years in Greensboro, NC. She loved this job and mastered her skills in the mental health field.

Barbara was also a Sunday School teacher, Director of Children's Church, an usher and a member of the Education Committee.

Barbara suffered a stroke at the age of 67 that changed life for her at that time. However, now, she is doing well with only a few negative side effects from the stroke.

Writing has been one of Barbara's passions for many years. She started pursuing this passion in the early 1970's. Her work has been published in the local paper as she recognized and honored the community. She decided to write because she felt that good deeds of people often go unnoticed, and she wanted to be an example for the creative and brilliant youth with whom she worked.

Today, Barbara is 75 years old and resides with her beloved and caring husband of 53 years, Connie Shuler. She is the proud mother of five children, 12 grandchildren and six great-grandchildren. She is a happy and devoted member of Mount Zion United Church of God and proclaims, "God has really blessed and healed my mind, body and soul."

Barbara is a compassionate and passionate woman who is driven by her love and appreciation of life and people.

Made in the USA
Columbia, SC
17 June 2024

36724345R00020